PHARMACOLOGIC EXPLANATION FOR THE OBSERVED GENDER DIFFERENCE IN RECOVERY FROM ANESTHESIA

ANESTHETIC PHARMACOLOGY 101 (US)

YEWANDE OKUNOREN-OYEKENU, DBAc

Copyright and Title

Title   Pharmacologic explanation for the observed gender difference in recovery from anesthesia

Subtitle   Anesthetic Pharmacology 101 (US)

ISBN   978-1-008-96632-1

Imprint/Publisher   Lulu.com

Copyright License   All Rights Reserved
Standard Copyright License

Copyright Holder   Yewande Okunoren Oyekenu

Copyright Year   2021

Contributors   By (author) Yewande Okunoren-Oyekenu
Photographs by Abidoba Oyekenu

Edition   Special edition

Edition Statement   This book is written to contribute to knowledge as part of the celebration of the 40th Birthday of Yewande Okunoren-Oyekenu and 16th Birthday of Abidoba Oyindamola Maria Oyekenu. It is dedicated to Foluseke Demilade Oyekenu. May his soul rest in peace.

DEDICATION

I dedicate this book to my late husband, Foluseke Demilade Oyekenu, who supported me during my research. May your soul rest in perfect peace.

ACKNOWLEDGMENTS

I am grateful to God Almighty for his mercies and my daughter's patience during my academic journey. Abidoba, I am happy to be a positive influence in your life.

My parents, Very Revd Dr. (Capt) Philip Adebayo and Mrs. Helen Olufunmilayo Okunoren, have supported me morally and financially. I am grateful to have you as my parents. My sisters, Abiodun, Adeseye, and Opeyemi, and their spouses, Adewale, Bamidele, and Olumide, have played an essential role in my life by taking care of my child whenever I have to conduct experimental work which disapproves of children in the laboratory. Thank you so much, and may God bless you and your family.

I thank the entire Okunoren and Oyekenu family, friends, and colleagues who have supported me during my research studies.

SYNOPSIS

This book is for healthcare professionals and the public interested in how anesthetic agents elicit their effects. It provides essential information on the influence of gender and ethnicity on the metabolism of general anesthetic agents. The impact of the type of surgery is also discussed, with a focus on recovery from anesthesia after rhinoplasty. Due to popular demand to explain my research results, I have written this book called Anesthetic Pharmacology 101 as guidance to a patient-centric approach to anesthesia practice and considerations for dosage regimen in a gender-wise and ethnic fashion for best results in recovery from general anesthetics. Anesthetic Pharmacology 102, an advanced pharmacokinetic study, is available on request as a PowerPoint presentation for educational purposes. I do hope you enjoy reading this book. Thank you.

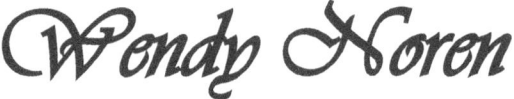

Wendy Noren

TABLE OF CONTENTS

CHAPTER 1

GENDER AND ETHNIC DIFFERENCES

IN RECOVERY FROM ANESTHESIA

Gender is a known factor in recovery from general anesthetics. Okunoren-Oyekenu *et al* (2014) reports such a difference, and proposes gender-based differences in pharmacokinetic profiles as explanation. Two main strata (20 black males and 20 black females) were considered, and written informed consents were obtained for both strata. Intravenous general anesthesia was induced with propofol or thiopental and maintained with inhalational agent halothane or isoflurane. Patient plasma samples were analyzed with high performance liquid chromatography (HPLC), for anesthetic agents before induction; at 10, 30 60, 180 mins after induction of anesthesia, and at recovery. The elimination half-life, mean resident time, and clearance measured in propofol patients maintained on halothane or isoflurane were 310.7 ± 138.4 min, 459.2 ± 199.4 min and 431.1 ± 154.1 ml/min, respectively for females versus 503.0 ± 312.2 min, 732.8 ± 448.3 min and 290.0 ± 157.8 ml/min for males. The corresponding values with thiopental induction were 148.0 ± 112.7 min, 220.9 ± 180.3 min and 544.6 ± 500.1 ml/min for females versus 76.8 ± 28.7 min, 115.4 ± 35.4 min and 533.7 ± 502.5 ml/min for males. Data was significantly different ($p<0.05$) across gender. The South-West Nigerian study concluded that gender differences in recovery from anesthetic agents is due to differences in pharmacokinetic profiles.

Drug-drug interactions and the route of administration of drugs may impact the observed gender differences in the Okunoren-Oyekenu *et al.* (2014) study. Their study made use of propofol or thiopental as intravenous induction and maintained anesthesia by inhalational anesthesia with isoflurane or halothane. Isoflurane and halothane may have affected the pharmacokinetics of propofol or thiopental anesthesia. However, the pharmacokinetics of halothane and isoflurane was not analyzed by their study, due to a lack of resources in low and middle-income countries.

Gender differences in the ability to tolerate pain stimulus have been reported both preclinically and clinically (Ellermeier *et al.*, 1995; Feine *et al.*, 1991; Gutiérrez Lombana & Gutiérrez Vidál, 2012). Variation in gender for binding to the μ (Op3) receptor leads to differences in the threshold for pain among gender (Zubeital *et al.*, 1999). The female patients in the Okunoren-Oyekenu *et al.* (2014) study had more post-operative backaches and headaches than the males. Overall, the females on thiopental anesthesia had more post-operative complications than the females on propofol anesthesia. Males had a better state at recovery than the females with the anesthetics studied. Due to an increase in the tendency to have lumbar lordosis, migraine, and headaches, women are more at risk of post-operative complications like backaches, headaches, and nausea (Ajuzieogu *et al.*, 2011; Murrie *et al.*, 2003; Stadler *et al.*, 2003).

Sedative premedication was omitted in the patients of the Okunoren-Oyekenu *et al.* (2014) study. According to Stadler *et al.* (2003), "female gender, non-smoking status, and general anesthesia increase both post-operative nausea and vomiting." Had sedative premedication been employed in their study of black patients, it is unsure if the pharmacokinetics of the anesthetics studied would have been different. Maurice-Szamburski *et al.* (2015) did not find any significance between sedative premedication with lorazepam and perioperative experience. During the post-operative period, Kim *et al.* (2017) did not find any significance between sedative premedication with midazolam and recovery. Additional studies are needed with respect to the effects of pre-operative drugs and smoking status on recovery from anesthesia.

Appropriate endotracheal-sized tubes were used for participants in the Okunoren-Oyekenu *et al.* (2014) study. Endotracheal tube intubation has been linked with post-operative sore throats and hoarseness, leading to post-operative sore throats been rated among the ten worst post-operative complications (Christensen *et al.*, 1994; Jaensson *et al.*, 2014; Loeser *et al.*, 1980 and Macario *et al.*, 1999). However, there are contradictory reports on gender-wise effects of endotracheal tube on sore throats (Canbay *et al.*, 2008; Myles *et al.*, 2001). Jaensson *et al.* (2014) studied endotracheal tube effects among gender and observed no gender difference in the incidence of post-operative sore throat and hoarseness, which may be attributed to using a reduced-sized endotracheal tube in women. However, Okunoren-Oyekenu *et al.* (2014) showed a gender-wise difference as female patients reported moderate to severe sore throats, unlike males who reported none to mild. This study by Okunoren-Oyekenu *et al.* (2014), therefore, is in agreement with the works of Myles *et al.* (2001), Ajuzieogu *et al.* (2011), and Fenta *et al.* (2020) that observed gender differences in post-operative sore throats incidence.

To make statistically significant conclusions in gender-wise comparative studies, the weight of the males and females of the research must be comparable. The results from Okunoren-Oyekenu *et al.* (2014) have satisfied the criteria required to make a gender-wise comparison. The average weight for participants was 65kg for females and 70kg for males. The 5kg variation among strata is expected as the average weight of females and males in the study demographic was represented by the Okunoren-Oyekenu *et al.* (2014) study. The anesthetic drugs were administered by weight (mg/kg) as a standard requirement, making their study results justifiable. However, other factors such as hormonal, neuroanatomical, and physiological differences among gender affect drug metabolism, resulting in the difference Okunoren-Oyekenu *et al.* (2014) have reported.

As far back as 2001, Ortolani, Conti, Sall, *et al.* (2001) reported that forty-five Black Africans of Senegalese ethnicity took a longer time to recover from propofol anesthesia when compared with an equivalent number of Caucasians of Italian background based on the evidence from a bispectral index of propofol metabolism. Within the same period, an Australian study by Myles *et al.* (2001) reported gender differences in two hundred and forty-one male patients and two hundred and twenty-two female patients undergoing surgery with propofol anesthesia. Female patients resulting from hormonal differences that impacted propofol anesthesia's metabolism were able to recover as measured by eye-opening and obeying commands but reported more post-operative complications (Myles *et al.* 2001). Researchers recognize gender and racial differences in metabolism. Several studies have been conducted afterward but with more focus on racial clinical parameters and fewer studies on racial pharmacokinetics and gender-based pharmacokinetic differences.

A few studies relating to racial differences reported that recovery from anesthesia among patients was more rapid in Caucasians, followed by Brazilians, and then Kenyans had the worst recovery of all three groups studied (Ortolani, O., Conti, A., Ngumi, *et al.,* 2004). When Chinese, Indian, Malaysia, and Caucasian patients were compared, Chinese and Caucasian patients recovered faster, Malaysians and Indians had a slower recovery, but Indians were having the most prolonged time recovering from anesthesia (Ortolani, Conti, Chani, *et al.,* 2004). Natarajan *et al.* (2011) compared fifty white and fifty black patients in Britain and obtained similar results with Ortolani, Conti, Sall, *et al.* (2001). Rather than providing a standard dose to all patients, the patients were anesthetized by racial requirement, which meant a lower propofol dose to initiate unconsciousness was required in blacks than in their white counterparts (Natarajan *et al.,* 2011). In the US, a comparison of fifteen black and twenty-eight white patients revealed differences among both groups with respect to their overall surgical experiences (Dos Santos Marques *et al.,* 2020). However, when post-operative pain among five hundred and eighty-five patients was analyzed by age and gender, there was no clinically significant difference despite younger adults reporting increased pain scores (Kanaan, 2021).

Puri *et al.* (2011) studied propofol pharmacokinetics in Indian patients, and the results obtained were 5,500ng/ml at 2min and 0ng/ml at 24hrs after induction of anesthesia for surgical procedures lasting two hours or less. It is not fully understood whether racial differences exist regarding the pharmacokinetics of the anesthetics studied. However, the critical fact is that a gender difference is widely reported across all ethnic groups so far studied as supported by female patients having more post-operative complications with anesthesia. More recently, pain sensitivity was observed among healthy females, thirty Chinese and thirty Indians, with female Indian participants exhibiting an increased sensitivity to pain than their Chinese co-participants (Ng, 2019).

Gender and ethnicity studies with respect to the pharmacokinetics of anesthetic agents are not fully established in developing countries (Choo, 2020; Puri *et al.,* 2011). While Puri *et al.* (2011) studied propofol pharmacokinetics in twenty-six Indian patients undergoing surgery for less than two hours, Okunoren-Oyekenu *et al.* (2014) performed an additional step of investigating differences in the pharmacokinetics of propofol and thiopental maintained with halothane or isoflurane by a gender-wise comparison of twenty black females and twenty black males undergoing surgery for nine hours or less. Studies to analyze the influence of ethnicity on the metabolism of drugs like anesthetic agents should be encouraged to enhance individualized dosage regimen.

CHAPTER 2

ETHNICITY AND RECOVERY FROM ANESTHESIA

AFTER RHINOPLASTY

In the previous chapter, ethnicity as defined by skin color and its impact on recovery from anesthesia was addressed. The influence of gender on recovery was also addressed. However, the type of surgery may also contribute to recovery from anesthesia. Patients in the Okunoren-Oyekenu *et al.* (2014) study was presented for various surgical procedures such as appendicectomy, dc rhinostomy, total laryngectomy, total thyroidectomy, exploratory laparatomy, tonsillectomy, herniorrhaphy, and mastectomy. Vascular complications, migraines, and headaches have been reported as some adverse events following non-surgical rhinoplasty (Benjamin *et al.*, 2020; Chen, Liu & Fan, 2016). While rhinoplasty may be achieved non-surgically, the focus of this review is surgical rhinoplasty under general anesthesia.

Humans have similar anatomy irrespective of race, but one fascinating ethnic variation is the nose due to differences in shape and size. The patients of the Okunoren-Oyekenu *et al.* (2014) study were black patients. Zhuang *et al.*, 2010 studied the use of personal protective equipment (PPE) among an ethnically diverse US workforce and observed a variation in the architecture of the nose. According to Zhuang *et al.* (2010), "African-Americans have statistically shorter, wider, and shallower noses than Caucasians." It was also revealed that noses of African descent weigh more than other races (Zhuang *et al.*, 2010). Based on these variations in width and weight, noses of African descent will likely require a longer duration of surgery for aesthetic purposes or improvement in breathing function compared with noses from other races.

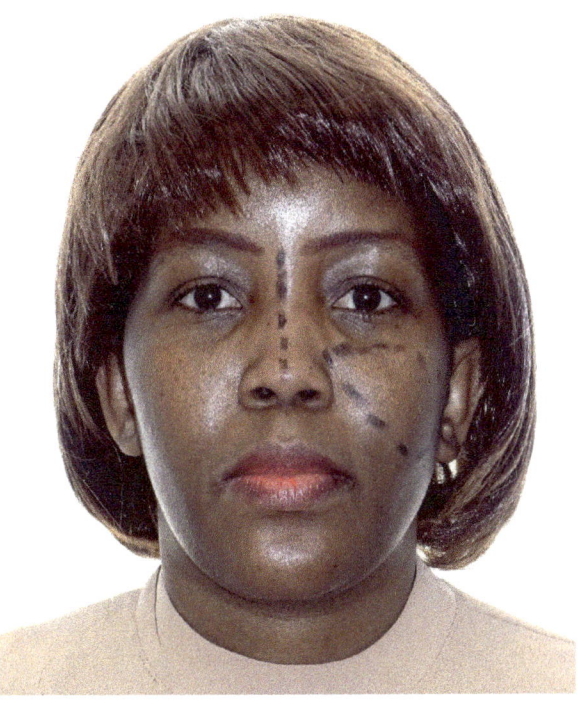

Figure 1. Example of an image of markings for facial surgery

Facial marking credit; the Author (Yewande Okunoren-Oyekenu).

Figure 1 shows a black female model (the author) display of facial markings for surgery.

It serves as an improvement over commonly available images in medical books due to variation in races of models presented for study. Black models should be encouraged to take part in the advertisement of reputable medical services and products. The author is happy to have her image in this book as she is also a commercial model for healthcare-related products. The author also has her image on the book's cover as an example of a facial half. She serves as a role model for black female scientists to promote healthcare services effectively when they have accurate product knowledge.

As ethnic differences have been studied and revealed to impact recovery from anesthesia, the type of transformation to the nose of patients also determines the duration of surgery and, in turn, duration of anesthesia leading to differences in recovery after rhinoplasty under exposure to general anesthesia. According to Gao *et al.* (2018), "compared with White women, East Asian women prefer a small, delicate, and less robust face, lower position of double eyelid, more obtuse nasofrontal angle, rounder nose tip, smaller tip projection, and slightly more retruded mandibular profile". Ramanadham (2021) reports that South Asian women comprise minority groups in plastic surgery practice in the US. With the kinds of transformation required to noses based on ethnic preferences and a shortage of female plastic surgeons from ethnic backgrounds, collaboration with surgeons in African and Asian countries should be encouraged to improve outcomes for these patients seeking westernization of their noses. The ethnic differences imply that training in rhinoplasty should be sensitive to ethnicity. Rhinoplasty and its impact on recovery from anesthesia should be carefully explained to patients as an individual experience instead of a standard recovery pattern due to variation in ethnicity (Villanueva *et al.*, 2019).

CHAPTER 3

POST-OPERATIVE PAIN MEASUREMENT

IN ANESTHESIA MANAGEMENT

Gender and ethnic differences in recovery from general anesthesia have been studied for several years. It has been widely established that there are differences in gender and ethnicity concerning recovery time from anesthesia. What has not been fully established is the pharmacologic explanation for these observed differences. When recruiting study participants for medical research, there is a tendency to exclude females due to concerns surrounding teratogenicity (congenital disabilities) and some ethical guidelines that automatically make women fall into the exclusion list. Of the 40 patients studied by Okunoren-Oyekenu et al. (2014), there was no case of mental impairment. Females on thiopental anesthesia experienced more postoperative complications than females on propofol anesthesia. The females in their study took a shorter time to recover from propofol than their male counterparts. (4 mins 40secs for females vs. 9mins 45secs for males at $P<0.05$). While with thiopental, the result obtained was reversed with females emerging more slowly (8min 55sec) than males 4mins 15secs after anesthesia. The recovery time was longer in females on thiopental anesthesia, 8 min 55 secs, compared with females on propofol, 4 mins 40 secs.

Some patients in their study had other postoperative complications in addition to regular nausea and vomiting, sore throat, headaches, and backaches reported by most patients (Okunoren-Oyekenu *et al.*, 2014). One patient on propofol complained of pain in the thigh (male patient 001M), while with thiopental anesthesia, other complications were general body pains (male patient 003M), shoulder pain (female patient 009F), excessive vomiting (female patient 011F and 020F) and dry mouth (female patient 011F). There was no record of the death of any patient in their study. The observed gender differences in recovery from propofol and thiopental (maintained on halothane or isoflurane) provided by the Okunoren-Oyekenu *et al.* (2014) study have been supported by the pharmacokinetic parameters obtained with laboratory analysis and corresponding clinical assessment. Gender comparison in recovery from anesthesia by this pharmacokinetic study has satisfied the need to explain the observed differences in gender and in black patients who fall within the group of reluctant patients to engage in research programs.

Observed clinical outcomes in patients have accompanied pharmacokinetic parameters in several studies. However, one area of concern is the measurement of pain scores, as this has been a study limitation in various research studies. Pain is subjective, and there are contradictory reports on pain scores across multiple research results due to patients providing scores because of psychologic or cultural influence. Gutiérrez Lombana & Gutiérrez Vidál (2012) observed that while male patients reported no pain or mild pain when asked by female medical staff, female patients, on the other hand, reported higher pain scores than their male counterparts when they were asked by male medical staff. Issues such as this lead to an overdose of pain medication if the patient has self-reported an actual score increase. Also, one patient's extreme pain can be described as mild pain by another patient depending on their pain threshold and tolerance, as observed in gender-wise comparative studies. Innovations similar to digital blood-glucose meters that can accurately measure pain levels as opposed to patient self-reported scores are needed in pain management.

Several studies have reported differences in gender with respect to recovery from anesthesia. Some studies observed gender differences in recovery as the ability to be discharged as measured by regaining consciousness and restoring the individual's pre-operative physiologic/healthy status (Eduardo *et al.*, 2016). Unfortunately, women are found to have worsened side effects from general anesthesia despite the enhanced ability to obey commands in the immediate post-operative period compared to their male counterparts (Ajuzieogu *et al.*, 2011). According to Myles *et al.* (2001), thirty-three percent of women versus sixteen percent of men experience post-operative complications such as post-operative nausea and vomiting, headaches, backaches, and sore throats. It implies that research should describe recovery from anesthesia with caution to avoid patients' early discharge, which may lead to the higher incidence of readmissions associated with post-operative complications (Kelly *et al.*, 2015; Kohlnhofer *et al.*, 2014). Anesthetic agents such as propofol are lipophilic (fat-loving); hence, patients that are obese are likely to experience worsened side effects such as nausea and vomiting.

The current general anesthetics used globally cause undesirable side effects; however, due to intricacies surrounding the approval of new or potential therapeutic agents, it has been challenging to create drugs that have specific target receptors and lesser side effects. Additional research on gender differences is needed to identify what factors cause these differences. Pharmacokinetic analysis of anesthetic agents can generate data such as concentration versus time curves, which may give insight into how differences in men and women arise rather than relying on eye-opening, obeying commands or pain scores as measurements. The Okunoren-Oyekenu *et al.* (2014) clinical and pharmacokinetic comparison is a tool in identifying the variation in the drug distribution of the anesthetics between the gender and its effects on recovery.

In conclusion, the type of disease, type of surgery, brain structure, and other patient characteristics also influence anesthetic agents' metabolism. Rhinoplasty has been addressed in this module as ethnic differences arise with the nose's shape and size, impacting surgery and anesthesia duration when a transformation is required. Non-surgical rhinoplasty may have advantages over surgical rhinoplasty; however, many patients have had to turn to unlicensed cosmetic surgeons due to a shortage of professional plastic surgeons (Ramanadham, 2021).

The COVID-19 pandemic may also impact the need for rhinoplasty due to face mask use, which is likely to cause damage to the nose, with healthcare workers being at greater risk due to prolonged use of masks in healthcare settings (Cabbarzade, 2020). With improvement in diversity and inclusion programs to increase the number of female plastic surgeons, there will be a reduction in complications from rhinoplasty when they are performed by licensed practitioners (Keane *et al.*, 2021; Ramanadham, 2021). Studies that measure the pharmacokinetics and clinical effects of alternative and improved general anesthetic agents by combining the influence of ethnicity, gender, age, obesity, drinking habit, and smoking status in the recovery from anesthesia are recommended. Prospective studies should also examine the role of brain damage on recovery from anesthesia. The next module in this course is Anesthetic Pharmacology 201, traumatic brain injury and its implication in anesthesia. Anesthetic Pharmacology 101 (this module) and Anesthetic Pharmacology 102 (for tutors) are required modules to ensure an adequate understanding of Anesthetic Pharmacology 201.

REFERENCES

Ajuzieogu, V.O., Amucheazi, A.O., Ezike, H.A. and Nwajiobi, C. (2011). Gender difference and quality of Recovery after general anaesthesia. *The Internet Journal of Anesthesiology*. 28.2.

Benjamin, M., McGregor, A., Yousif, S., Shaikh, D., & Reish, R. G. (2020). Entrapment Neuropathy Causing Persistent Headache Symptoms after Nonsurgical Rhinoplasty. *Plastic and reconstructive surgery. Global open*, *8*(12), e3209.

Cabbarzade, C. (2020). A Practical Way to Prevent Nose and Cheek Damage Due to the Use of N95 Masks in the COVID-19 Pandemic, *Aesthetic Surgery Journal*, 40(10), NP608–NP610.

Canbay, O., Celebi, N; Sahin, A; Celiker, V., Ozgen, S. and Aypar, U. (2008). Ketamine gargle for attenuating post operative sore throats *British Journal of Anesthesia* 100.4; p490 – 493.

Chen, Q., Liu, Y., & Fan, D. (2016). Serious Vascular Complications after Nonsurgical Rhinoplasty: A Case Report. *Plastic and reconstructive surgery. Global open*, *4*(4), e683.

Choo, V. (2020). The State of Anesthesia Practice in Sub-Saharan Africa: Statistics, Case Studies, and Ways Forward. The University of Texas South Western Medical Center, Thesis.

Christensen, A.M; Willemoes – Larsen, H; Lundby, L and Jakobsen, K.B. (1994). Postoperative throat camplaints after tracheal intubation. *British Journal of Anaesthesia* 73; p786 – 787.

Christensen, J.H; Andreasen, F and Jansen, J.A. (2011). Influence of Age and Sex on the pharmacokinetics of thiopentone. *Br J Anaesth* 53. 11:1189 – 1195.

Dos Santos Marques, I.C., Herbey, I.I., Theiss, L.M., Hollis, R.H., Knight, S.J., Davis, T.C., Fouad, M. & Chu, D.I. (2020). Understanding the Surgical Experience for African-Americans and Caucasians With Enhanced Recovery. *Journal of Surgical Research*, 250; p.2-22.

Eduardo, T. M., Fábio, C. O. L., Bernardo, R.N., Gustavo, F.P.S., Nathália V. & Laís, H.C.N. (2016). Quality of recovery from anesthesia of patients undergoing balanced or total intravenous general anesthesia. Prospective randomized clinical trial, Journal of Clinical Anesthesia, 35; p369-375.

Ellermeier, W. and Westphal, W. (1995). Gender differences in pain ratings and pupil reactions to painful pressure stimuli. *Pain* 61; p435 -439.

Feine, J.S; Bushnell, M.C; Miron, D. and Duncan, G.H. (1991). Sex differences in the perception of noxious heat stimuli. *Pain* 44; p255 – 262.

Fenta, E.,Teshome, D., Melaku, D. & Tesfaw, A. (2020). Incidence and factors associated with postoperative sore throat for patients undergoing surgery under general anesthesia with endotracheal intubation at Debre Tabor General Hospital, North central Ethiopia: A cross-sectional study. *International Journal of Surgery Open*, 25; p.1-5.

Gao. Y., Niddam, J., Noel, W., Hersant, B. & Meningaud, J. P. (2018). Comparison of aesthetic facial criteria between Caucasian and East Asian female populations: An esthetic surgeon's perspective, *Asian Journal of Surgery*, 41(1); p4-11.

Gutiérrez Lombana, W, & Gutiérrez Vidál, S. E. (2012). Pain and gender differences. A clinical approach. *Colombian Journal of Anestesiology*, 40(3); p207-212.

Jaensson, M., Gupta, A. & Nilsson, U. (2014). Gender differences in sore throat and hoarseness following endotracheal tube or laryngeal mask airway: a prospective study. *BMC Anesthesiol* 14(56).

Kanaan, S.F., Melton, B.L., Waitman, L.R., Simpson, M.H. and Sharma, N.K. (2021), The effect of age and gender on acute postoperative pain and function following lumbar spine surgeries. *Physiother Res Int*, 26.

Keane, A. M., Larson, E. L., Santosa, K. B., Vannucci, B., Waljee, J. F., Tenenbaum, M., Mackinnon, S. E. & Snyder-Warwick, A. K. (2021). Women in Leadership and Their Influence on the Gender Diversity of Academic Plastic Surgery Programs, *Plastic and Reconstructive Surgery*, 147(3); p.516-526.

Kelly, K.N., Iannuzzi, J.C., Aquina, C.T., Probst, C.P., Noyes, K., Monson, J.R.T. and Fleming, F.J. (2015). Timing of Discharge: a key to Understanding the Reason for Readmission after Colorectal Surgery. *J Gastrointest Surg* 19; p418-428.

Kim, M. H., Kim, M. S., Lee, J. H., Seo, J. H., & Lee, J. R. (2017). Can quality of recovery be enhanced by premedication with midazolam?: A prospective, randomized, double-blind study in females undergoing breast surgery. *Medicine*, *96*(7), e6107.

Kohlnhofer, B.M., Tevis, S. E., Weber, S. M. & Kennedy, G. D. (2014). Multiple complications and short length of stay are associated with postoperative readmissions, *The American Journal of Surgery*, 207(4); p.449-456.

Loeser, E.A., Bennett, G.M., Orr D.L. and Stanlrey, T.H. (1980). Reduction of postoperative sore throat with new endotracheal tube cuffs. *Anesthesiology*. 52; p257.

Marcario, A. Weinger, M., Carney, S. and Kim, A. (1999). Which clinical anaesthesia outcome are important to avoid? The perspective of patients. *Anesth Analg.* 89; p652 – 658.

Maurice-Szamburski A, Auquier P, Viarre-Oreal V, *et al.* (2015). Effect of Sedative Premedication on Patient Experience After General Anesthesia: A Randomized Clinical Trial. *JAMA*, 313(9); p916–925

Murrie, V. Dixon, A., Hollingworth, W; Wilson, H and Doyle, T. (2003). Lumbar lordosis: study of patients with and without low back pain. *Clinical Anatomy*, 16; p144 – 147.

Myles P.S., McLeod A.D., Hunt J.O., and Fletcher, H. (2001). Sex differences in speed of emergence and quality of recovery after anaesthesia; cohort study. *British Medical Journal,* 322; p710-711.

Natarajan, A., Strandvik, G.F., Pattanayak, R., Chakithandy, S., Passalacqua, A.M., Lewis, C.M. and Morley, A.P. (2011). Effect of ethnicity on the hypnotic and cardiovascular characteristics of propofol induction. *Anaesthesia*, 66; p15-19.

Ng, T. S. (2019). Racial differences in experimental pain sensitivity and conditioned pain modulation: a study of Chinese and Indians. *Journal of pain research, 12,* 2193–2200.

Okunoren-Oyekenu, Y., Sanusi, A., *et al.* (2014). Gender comparison of recovery from intravenous and inhalational anaesthetics among adult patients in South-West Nigeria (1064.3). *The FASEB Journal, 28.*

Ortolani, O., Conti, A., Chan, Y. K., Sie, M. Y., & Ong, G. S. Y. (2004). Comparison of Propofol Consumption and Recovery Time in Caucasians from Italy, with Chinese, Malays and Indians from Malaysia. *Anaesthesia and Intensive Care, 32*(2); p250–255.

Ortolani, O., Conti, A., Ngumi, Z.W., Texeira, L., Olang, P., Amani, I. & Medrado, V.C. (2004). Ethnic differences in propofol and fentanyl response: a comparison among Caucasians, Kenyan Africans and Brazillians. *European Journal of Anesthesiology*, 21(4); p314-319.

Ortolani, O., Conti, A., Sall, B., Salleras, J., Diouf, E., Kane, O., Roberts, S. & Novelli, G. (2001). The recovery of Senegalese African Blacks from intravenous anesthesia with propofol and remifentanil is slower than that of Caucasians. *Anesthesia & Analgesia*, 93(5); p1222-1226.

Puri, A., Mehdi, B. Panda, N.B. Puri, G.D. and Dhawan, S. (2011). Estimation of Pharmacokinetics of propofol in Indian patients by HPLC method. *J. Analy Bioanal Techniques*. 2.2: 1000120.

Ramanadham, S. R. (2021). South Asian Women: The Unexpected Minority in Plastic Surgery, *Plastic and Reconstructive Surgery*: 147(3); p.792-794.

Stadler, M., Bardiau, F., Seidel, L., Albert, A. and Boogaerts, J.G. (2003). Difference in risk factors for post operative nausea and vomiting. *Anesthesiology*. 98; p.46 – 52.

Villanueva. N. L., Afrooz, P.N., Carboy, J.A., Rohrich, R.J. (2019). Nasal Analysis: Considerations for Ethnic Variation. *Plast Reconstr Surg.* 143(6); 1179e-1188e.

Zhuang, Z., Landsittel, D., Benson, S., Roberge, R. & Shaffer, R. (2010). Facial Anthropometric Differences among Gender, Ethnicity, and Age Groups, *The Annals of Occupational Hygiene*, 54(4); p.391–402.

Zubieta, J.K., Dannals, R.F. and Frost J.J. (1999). Gender and age influences on human brain mu-opioid receptor binding measured by PET. *Am J Psychiatry*. 156; p.842 – 848.

SUGGESTED READING

Berchtold, V., Stofferin, H., Moriggl, B., Brenner, E., Pauzenberger, R. & Konschake, M. (2017). The supraorbital region revisited: An anatomic exploration of the neuro-vascular bundle with regard to frontal migraine headache, *Journal of Plastic, Reconstructive & Aesthetic Surgery*, 70(9); p.1171-1180.

Campesi, I., Fois, M. and Franconi, F. (2013). Sex and Gender Aspects in Anesthetics and Pain Madication. In: Regitz-Zagrosek V. (eds). Sex and Gender Differences in Pharmacology. Handbook of Experimental Pharmacology, vol 214. Springer, Berlin, Heidelberg.

Dawidowicz, A.L., Kalitynski, R. and Fijalkowska, A. (2003), Free and bound propofol concentrations in human cerebrospinal fluid. British Journal of Clinical Pharmacology, 56: 545-550

Gilberto C., Roberto, T., Massimo T., Massimo T. and Bonfigli, A. (2001). Fast, Simple and Cost – effective determination of Thiopental in human plasma by a new HPLC technique. *Clinical Chimica Acta* 305; 41 – 45

Hoymork, S.C. and Raeder, J. (2005). Why do women wake up faster than men from propofol anaesthesia. *British Journal of Anaesthesia*. 95.5: p657 - 633.

Misal, U. S., Joshi, S. A., & Shaikh, M. M. (2016). Delayed recovery from anesthesia: A postgraduate educational review. *Anesthesia, essays and researches*, *10*(2); p164–172.

Xavier C., Smet, E., Lantsoght, K., Salvi, J., Bolon- Larger, M., and Boulieu. (2007). A rapid and simple HPLC method for the analysis of propofol in biological fluids. *Journal of Pharmaceutical and Biomedical Analysis* 44; p680-682

BIRTHDAY WISHES

16TH AND 40TH BIRTHDAYS OF ABIDOBA AND YEWANDE
JULY 2021

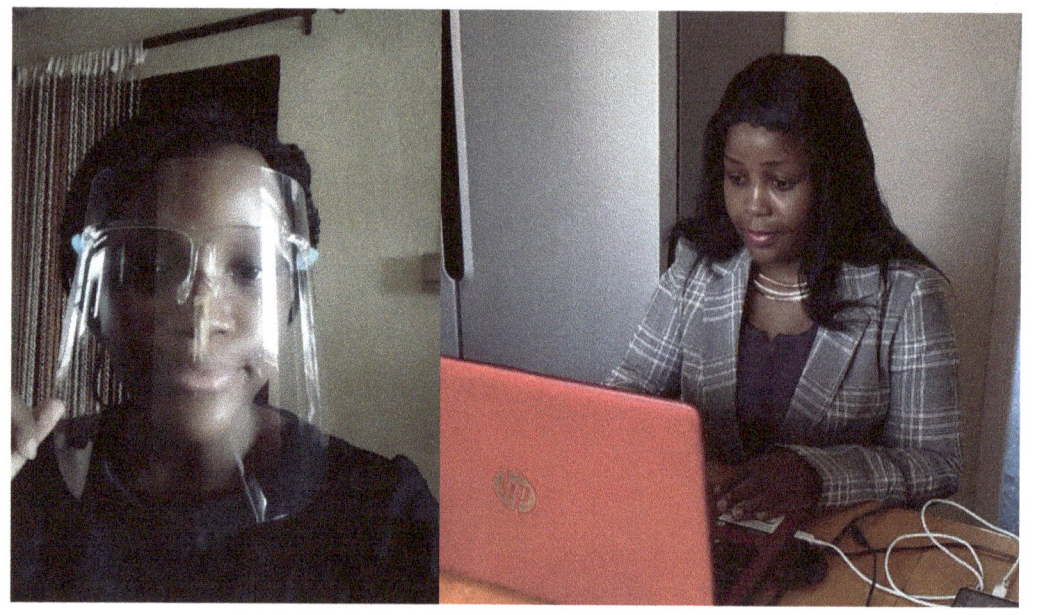

-

HAPPY BIRTHDAY ABIDOBA AND YEWANDE

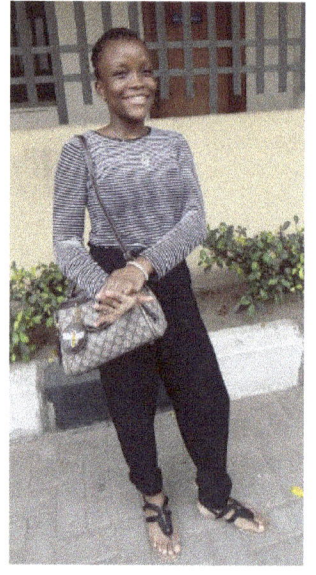 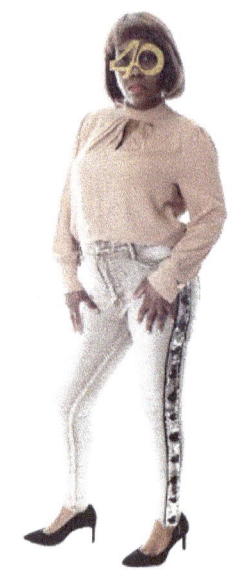

ORIKI ILE OKUNOREN/ THE OKUNOREN FAMILY

Ọmọ olóbì kan wókórótìró

Ọmọ olóbì kan wòkòròtìrò

Èyí tó bá je tení á wò sí òpò ẹní

Èyí tí ò bá jé tení á wò sínú igbó

Ẹranko búburú a má rohún mujẹ

Ọmọ akénigbó kẹrù kó ba ará òdàn

Ọmọ èlúkú mẹndẹ́n mẹndẹ́n ìmùlẹ̀

afẹ̀lẹ̀jà

Ọmọ asánipórìkì porìkí ẹsẹ̀

Ọmọ erín ó fọnmú

Erín báà fọnmú

O ṣe dẹ ní yẹn òkè déyìn

Ọmọ ẹyínta

Ọmọ ẹlègbèrẹ n òjé

Ọmọ asọrín sómọ

Ọmọ Àkárìgbò Kábíèsí rẹ o

Ọmọ ọwá n mí tìtì

Ọmọ Àkárìgbò Rẹ́mọ

Oríkí fun Abídoba /The Oyekenu Family

Òmọ àdó, àdó bàbà,

ògèdè làdó jẹ,

ẹ mámà bẹ́ ògèdè àdó ànù,

Ọmọ atẹ́ní wíjọ kí wẹ́wẹ̀wẹ́ òrọ̀ má ba

gbòn dànùù ọ

Ọmọ olóbì wówó tírí wó,

Ọmọ olobì wòwò tírí wò.

È tó fẹ́ní a wò sápò ẹ́ní,

èyí tí ò fẹ́ ní a wọ̀ sínú igbó

　Ọmọ ẹranko a fí jẹ

　Ọmọ ìta agada, ó ṣubú níta agada

　Ó fẹ nu gbé ítan olúbẹ̀

Birthday Messages for Abidoba

Happy birthday to my darling Abidoba.
As you become a lady, may you be exceptional in all your endeavors, may you have peace of mind. You would be a blessing to your generation. You shall live to proclaim the greatness of the Lord in the land of the living. As you have met my expectations for you and even surpassed, may the Lord also meet all your expectations.
Many happy returns my darling. Congratulations.
From Dr. Damilola Oyekenu

From the day you were born to this present time, everytime I look at you, I see the spitting image of my brother #smiles. As you celebrate another birthday, Abidoba I wish you a long, healthy, happy and a beautiful life.
May you be a source of joy and pride to us all.
Happy 16th birthday to you darling #kisses.
From Kunbi Lalude (Nee Oyekenu)

Abidoba, your light will never be dim.
Your strength will not be weary to attain better height. Continue to bask in the glory of God. Keep on flourishing even as you celebrate your new age!
Happy birthday my dear niece.
From Enitan Olateju (Nee Oyekenu)

1st July, 2021.

My dear granddaughter Maria Abidoba Oyekenu, I hope that your birthday is every bit as darling as you are. May it be filled with unparalleled happiness and a lifetime's worth of laughter and love. Happy birthday to the world's greatest granddaughter!

You always manage to fill my life with your positivity and love. I hope that you receive it back ten-fold on your special day. May you have a blessed day, and more importantly, may your presents be just as plentiful as your love is.

Your determination and strength inspire me, but it is your unconditional love that warms my soul. You are unbelievably precious to me, and I hope that your birthday is everything you want it to be.

HAPPY BIRTHDAY MARIA.

From Grandpa Okunoren
Very Revd Dr Capt Philip Adebayo Okunoren

From: Grandma
To: Abidoba Maria Oyekenu.

Happy.   16th   Birthday   to   my   highly.
esteemed Grand Daughter. I wish you Long Life,
Good health best of everything in nearest future.
 As you step on the ladder of Adulthood, may the
Lord give you the Grace to make excellent
achievements.
Your journeys in life will not be coupled with
sorrow.
The Almighty God will be your Refuge and He will
make you a Role Model and A Game Changer in
your generation.
The Blood of Jesus will always avail for you
because you are a Covenant Child.
 Happy Birthday my Sweetie Pie., Enjoy this Natal
Celebration to the Glory of God.
Much Love:
Grandma, Helen 'Funmi Okunoren

Birthday Messages for Yewande

15th July, 2021...

Happy 40th Birthday Anniversary to you my darling daughter Dr Yewande Omowunmi Okunoren-Oyekenu.

May you forever sparkle and shine like the star that you are.
Happy birthday my princess!
We wish you a birthday that is as beautiful, incredible, and unique as you are. Happy birthday daughter of Zion!
May your day be as bright as your smile and as lovely as you. Happy birthday my dear daughter!

 May each day of your year ahead be wonderful, at least as wonderful as the person you are, and bring the same joy to your heart as you do to all those around you. A very special happy birthday to you. Happy birthday to a VIP in my life! on your special day! REMAIN BLESSED!

From Daddy
Very Revd Dr Capt Philip Adebayo Okunoren

From Mother to daughter

My lovely daughter, I can't express the feelings I had, when for the first time I took you in my arms at around 10:50p.m .on 15th July, 1981. at the Military Hospital, Yaba, Lagos, Nigeria.
Your birthday is always a very special day for me.
My princess, today you are marking a milestone of 40 years in the Presence of God.
Happy birthday my little angel! ...
I thank the Lord for the Challenges you passed through which He turned to your pillars of Support, Victory and endless testimonies.
The Grace, Favour, Goodness and Mercies of the Lord shall be your portion all the days of your life in Jesus Name.
May the Holy Spirit continue to order your footsteps and make you a recipient of God's Covenant Blessings.
Wish you the Best of everything in Life.
Happy Birthday to the Lord's Chosen, I am proud of You.
Have a wonderful and remarkable Celebration.
Lots and Lots of Love:
Your Mum,
Mrs. Helen' Funmi Okunoren.

ABOUT THE TRANSLATOR

Abidoba Oyekenu is a technical science major interested in Astronomy, Aerospace and Mechanical Engineering. She had her primary education at Hazel Primary school, Leicester, UK and got an award for excellence in astronomy assignment. Abidoba started her secondary education at Hamilton College, Leicester UK before transferring to Rainbow College. She has translated her mother's book in healthcare to French and Spanish versions and hopes to add other languages to the list. This would improve communication in healthcare service, as well as the physician-patient experience when doctors can use digital health technology to translate patient's local language to English. Healthcare workers in non-English speaking regions will also have access to life-saving information for patients when their medical books are written in their local language.

ABOUT THE AUTHOR

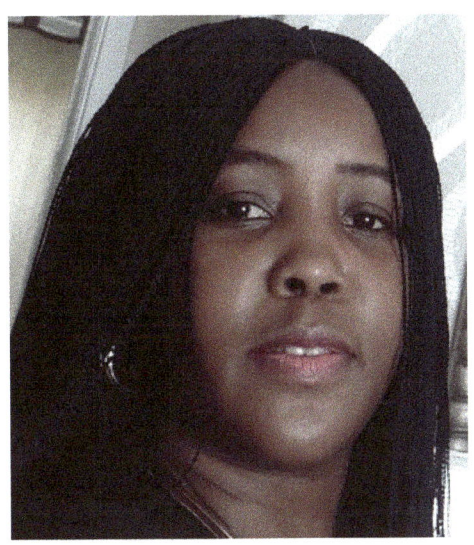

Yewande Okunoren-Oyekenu is a neuroscience researcher interested in healthcare innovations, trauma, neonatal brain repair, anesthesia, and pain management. She has a B.Sc. in Biochemistry from the Olabisi Onabanjo University, Nigeria, and an M.Sc. in Pharmacology and Therapeutics with a specialization in Pharmacokinetics from the University of Ibadan, Nigeria. Her Doctorate career started at the University of Leicester, UK, where she studied Cell Physiology and Pharmacology with a Neuroscience specialization before transferring to California Intercontinental University for a Doctorate of Business Administration in Healthcare Management and Leadership. She bridges the gap between medical research and industry to ensure the rapid translation of research results to benefit societal needs. She serves as an Advisory Board Member for healthcare organizations and encourages ages 9-18 to engage in STEM careers. Yewande was awarded a prize from the British Pharmacological Society for the best education poster presented at Pharmacology 2019, which has inspired her to make the subject anesthetic pharmacology easy to understand.